Pegan Main Courses and Side Dish Cookbook

A Collection of Easy Recipes for your Daily Tasty Meals

Kimberly Solis

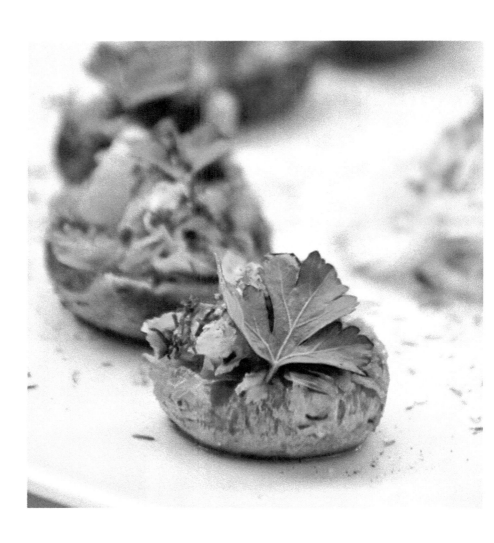

Table of Contents

Nachos

Preparation Time: 5 Minutes

Cooking Time: 10 Minutes

Servings: 4

Ingredients:

- 4-ounce restaurant-style corn tortilla chips

- 1 medium green onion, thinly sliced (about 1 tbsp.)

- 1 (4 ounces) package finely crumbled feta cheese

- 1 finely chopped and drained plum tomato

- 2 tbsp Sun-dried tomatoes in oil, finely chopped

- 2 tbsp Kalamata olives

Directions:

1. Mix an onion, plum tomato, oil, sun-dried tomatoes, and olives in a small bowl.

2. Arrange the tortillas chips on a microwavable plate in a single layer topped evenly with cheese—microwave on high for one minute.

3. Rotate the plate half turn and continue microwaving until the cheese is bubbly. Spread the tomato mixture over the chips and cheese and enjoy.

Nutrition:

Calories: 140

Carbs: 19g

Fat: 7g

Protein: 2g

Stuffed Celery

Preparation Time: 15 Minutes

Cooking Time: 20 Minutes

Servings: 3

Ingredients:

- Olive oil

- 1 clove garlic, minced

- 2 tbsp Pine nuts

- 2 tbsp dry-roasted sunflower seeds

- ¼ cup Italian cheese blend, shredded

- 8 stalks celery leaves

- 1 (8-ounce) fat-free cream cheese

- Cooking spray

Directions:

1. Sauté garlic and pine nuts over a medium setting for the heat until the nuts are golden brown. Cut off the wide base and tops from celery.

2. Remove two thin strips from the round side of the celery to create a flat surface.

3. Mix Italian cheese and cream cheese in a bowl and spread into cut celery stalks.

4. Sprinkle half of the celery pieces with sunflower seeds and a half with the pine nut mixture. Cover mixture and let stand for at least 4 hours before eating.

Nutrition:

Calories: 64

Carbs: 2g

Fat: 6g

Protein: 1g

Butternut Squash Fries

Preparation Time: 5 Minutes

Cooking Time: 10 Minutes

Servings: 2

Ingredients:

- 1 Butternut squash
- 1 tbsp Extra virgin olive oil
- ½ tbsp Grapeseed oil
- 1/8 tsp Sea salt

Directions:

1. Remove seeds from the squash and cut into thin slices. Coat with extra virgin olive oil and grapeseed oil. Add a sprinkle of salt and toss to coat well.

2. Arrange the squash slices onto three baking sheets and bake for 10 minutes until crispy.

Nutrition:

Calories: 40

Carbs: 10g

Fat: 0g

Protein: 1g

Dried Fig Tapenade

Preparation Time: 5 Minutes

Cooking Time: 0 Minutes

Servings: 1

Ingredients:

- 1 cup Dried figs

- 1 cup Kalamata olives

- ½ cup Water

- 1 tbsp Chopped fresh thyme

- 1 tbsp extra virgin olive oil

- ½ tsp Balsamic vinegar

Directions:

1. Prepare figs in a food processor until well chopped, add water, and continue processing to form a paste.

2. Add olives and pulse until well blended. Add thyme, vinegar, and extra virgin olive oil and pulse until very smooth. Best served with crackers of your choice.

Nutrition:

Calories: 249

Carbs: 64g

Fat: 1g

Protein: 3g

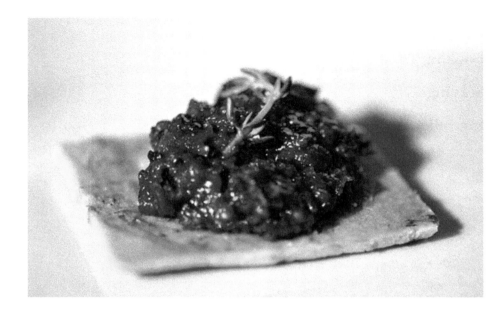

Speedy Sweet Potato Chips

Preparation Time: 15 Minutes

Cooking Time: 0 Minutes

Servings: 4

Ingredients:

- 1 large Sweet potato
- 1 tbsp Extra virgin olive oil
- Salt

Directions:

1. 300°F preheated oven. Slice your potato into nice, thin slices that resemble fries.

2. Toss the potato slices with salt and extra virgin olive oil in a bowl. Bake for about one hour, flipping every 15 minutes until crispy and browned.

Nutrition:

Calories: 150

Carbs: 16g

Fat: 9g

Protein: 1g

Nachos with Hummus

Preparation Time: 15 Minutes

Cooking Time: 20 Minutes

Servings: 4

Ingredients:

- 4 cups salted pita chips
- 1 (8 oz.) red pepper (roasted)
- Hummus
- 1 tsp Finely shredded lemon peel
- ¼ cup Chopped pitted Kalamata olives
- ¼ cup crumbled feta cheese
- 1 plum (Roma) tomato, seeded, chopped
- ½ cup chopped cucumber
- 1 tsp Chopped fresh oregano leaves

Directions:

1. 400°F preheated oven. Arrange the pita chips on a heatproof platter and drizzle with hummus.

2. Top with olives, tomato, cucumber, and cheese and bake until warmed through. Sprinkle lemon zest and oregano and enjoy while it's hot.

Nutrition:

Calories: 130

Carbs: 18g

Fat: 5g

Protein: 4g

Hummus and Olive Pita Bread

Preparation Time: 5 Minutes

Cooking Time: 0 Minutes

Servings: 3

Ingredients:

- 7 pita bread cut into 6 wedges each

- 1 (7 ounces) container plain hummus

- 1 tbsp Greek vinaigrette

- ½ cup Chopped pitted Kalamata olives

Directions:

1. Spread the hummus on a serving plate—Mix vinaigrette and olives in a bowl and spoon over the hummus. Enjoy with wedges of pita bread.

Nutrition:

Calories: 225

Carbs: 40g

Fat: 5g

Protein: 9g

Roast Asparagus

Preparation Time: 15 Minutes

Cooking Time: 5 Minutes

Servings: 4

Ingredients:

- 1 tbsp Extra virgin olive oil (1 tablespoon)
- 1 medium lemon
- ½ tsp Freshly grated nutmeg
- ½ tsp black pepper
- ½ tsp Kosher salt

Directions:

2. Warm the oven to 500°F. Put the asparagus on an aluminum foil and drizzle with extra virgin olive oil, and toss until well coated.

3. Roast the asparagus in the oven for about five minutes; toss and continue roasting until browned. Sprinkle the roasted asparagus with nutmeg, salt, zest, and pepper.

Nutrition:

Calories: 123

Carbs: 5g

Fat: 11g

Protein: 3g

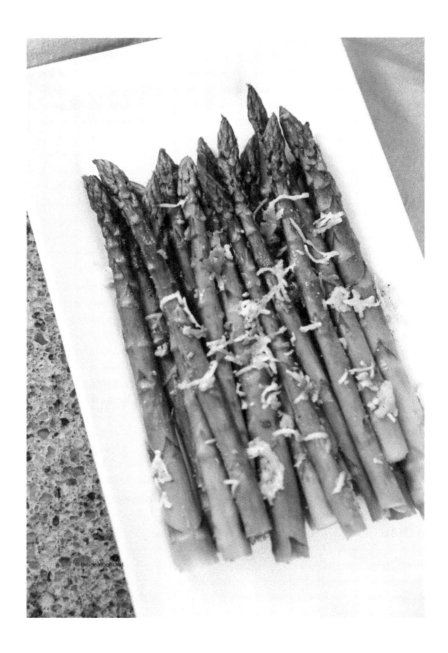

Chicken Kale Wraps

Preparation Time: 10 Minutes

Cooking Time: 10 Minutes

Servings: 4

Ingredients:

- 4 kale leaves
- 4 oz chicken fillet
- ½ apple
- 1 tablespoon butter
- ¼ teaspoon chili pepper
- ¾ teaspoon salt
- 1 tablespoon lemon juice
- ¾ teaspoon dried thyme

Directions:

1. Chop the chicken fillet into small cubes. Then mix up the chicken with chili pepper and salt.

2. Heat butter in the skillet. Add chicken cubes. Roast them for 4 minutes.

3. Meanwhile, chop the apple into small cubes and add to the chicken. Mix up well.

4. Sprinkle the ingredients with lemon juice and dried thyme. Cook them for 5 minutes over medium-high heat.

5. Fill the kale leaves with the hot chicken mixture and wrap.

Nutrition:

Calories 106

Fat 5.1

Fiber 1.1

Carbs 6.3

Protein 9

Tomato Triangles

Preparation Time: 10 Minutes

Cooking Time: 0 Minutes

Servings: 6

Ingredients:

- 6 corn tortillas
- 1 tablespoon cream cheese
- 1 tablespoon ricotta cheese
- ½ teaspoon minced garlic
- 1 tablespoon fresh dill, chopped
- 2 tomatoes, sliced

Directions:

1. Cut every tortilla into 2 triangles. Then mix up cream cheese, ricotta cheese, minced garlic, and dill.

2. Spread 6 triangles with cream cheese mixture.

3. Then place the sliced tomato on them and cover with remaining tortilla triangles. Serve.

Nutrition:

Calories 71

Fat 1.6

Fiber 2.1

Carbs 12.8

Protein 2.3

Zaatar Fries

Preparation Time: 10 Minutes

Cooking Time: 35 Minutes

Servings: 5

Ingredients:

- 1 teaspoon Zaatar spices

- 3 sweet potatoes

- 1 tablespoon dried dill

- 1 teaspoon salt

- 3 teaspoons sunflower oil

- ½ teaspoon paprika

Directions:

1. Pour water into the crockpot. Cut the sweet potatoes into fries.

2. Line the baking tray with parchment. Place the layer of the sweet potato in the tray.

3. Sprinkle the vegetables with dried dill, salt, and paprika. Then sprinkle sweet potatoes with Za'atar and mix up well with the help of the fingertips.

4. Sprinkle the sweet potato fries with sunflower oil—Preheat the oven to 375F.

5. Bake the sweet potato fries within 35 minutes. Stir the fries every 10 minutes.

Nutrition:

Calories 28

Fat 2.9

Fiber 0.2

Carbs 0.6

Protein 0.2

Summertime Vegetable Chicken Wraps

Preparation Time: 15 Minutes

Cooking Time: 0 Minutes

Servings: 4

Ingredients:

- 2 cups cooked chicken, chopped

- ½ English cucumbers, diced

- ½ red bell pepper, diced

- ½ cup carrot, shredded

- 1 scallion, white and green parts, chopped

- ¼ cup plain Greek yogurt

- 1 tablespoon freshly squeezed lemon juice

- ½ teaspoon fresh thyme, chopped

- Pinch of salt

- Pinch of ground black pepper

- 4 multigrain tortillas

Directions:

1. Take a medium bowl and mix in chicken, red bell pepper, cucumber, carrot, yogurt, scallion, lemon juice, thyme, sea salt and pepper.

2. Mix well.

3. Spoon one quarter of chicken mix into the middle of the tortilla and fold the opposite ends of the tortilla over the filling.

4. Roll the tortilla from the side to create a snug pocket.

5. Repeat with the remaining ingredients and serve.

6. Enjoy!

Nutrition:

Calories: 278

Fat: 4g

Carbohydrates: 28g

Protein: 27g

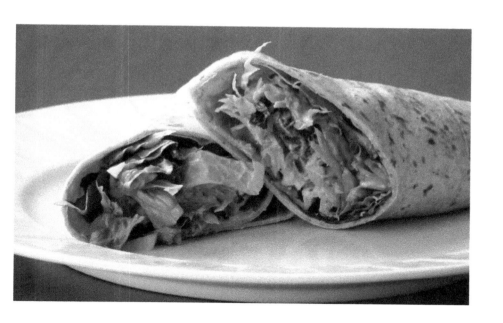

Premium Roasted Baby Potatoes

Preparation Time: 10 Minutes

Cooking Time: 35 Minutes

Servings: 4

Ingredients:

- 2 pounds new yellow potatoes, scrubbed and cut into wedges

- 2 tablespoons extra virgin olive oil

- 2 teaspoons fresh rosemary, chopped

- 1 teaspoon garlic powder

- 1 teaspoon sweet paprika

- ½ teaspoon sea salt

- ½ teaspoon freshly ground black pepper

Directions:

1. Pre-heat your oven to 400 degrees Fahrenheit.

2. Take a large bowl and add potatoes, olive oil, garlic, rosemary, paprika, sea salt and pepper.

3. Spread potatoes in single layer on baking sheet and bake for 35 minutes.

4. Serve and enjoy!

Nutrition:

Calories: 225

Fat: 7g

Carbohydrates: 37g

Protein: 5g

Tomato and Cherry Linguine

Preparation Time: 10 Minutes

Cooking Time: 15 Minutes

Servings: 4

Ingredients:

- 2 pounds cherry tomatoes
- 3 tablespoons extra virgin olive oil
- 2 tablespoons balsamic vinegar
- 2 teaspoons garlic, minced
- Pinch of fresh ground black pepper
- ¾ pound whole-wheat linguine pasta
- 1 tablespoon fresh oregano, chopped
- ¼ cup feta cheese, crumbled

Directions:

1. Pre-heat your oven to 350 degrees Fahrenheit.
2. Take a large bowl and add cherry tomatoes, 2 tablespoons olive oil, balsamic vinegar, garlic, pepper and toss.
3. Spread tomatoes evenly on baking sheet and roast for 15 minutes.

4. While the tomatoes are roasting, cook the pasta according to the package instructions and drain the paste into a large bowl.

5. Toss pasta with 1 tablespoon olive oil.

6. Add roasted tomatoes (with juice) and toss.

7. Serve with topping of oregano and feta cheese.

8. Enjoy!

Nutrition:

Calories: 397

Fat: 15g

Carbohydrates: 55g

Protein: 13g

Mediterranean Zucchini Mushroom Pasta

Preparation Time: 10 Minutes

Cooking Time: 10 Minutes

Servings: 4

Ingredients:

- ½ pound pasta
- 2 tablespoons olive oil
- 6 garlic cloves, crushed
- 1 teaspoon red chili
- 2 spring onions, sliced
- 3 teaspoons rosemary
- 1 large zucchini, cut in half
- 5 large portabella mushrooms
- 1 can tomatoes
- 4 tablespoons Parmesan cheese
- Fresh ground black pepper

Directions:

1. Cook the pasta.

2. Take a large-sized frying pan and place it over medium heat.

3. Add oil and allow the oil to heat up.

4. Add garlic, onion and chili and sauté for a few minutes until golden.

5. Add zucchini, rosemary and mushroom and sauté for a few minutes.

6. Increase the heat to medium-high and add tinned tomatoes to the sauce until thick.

7. Drain your boiled pasta and transfer to serving platter.

8. Pour the tomato mix on top and mix using tongs.

9. Garnish with Parmesan and freshly ground black pepper.

10. Enjoy!

Nutrition:

Calories: 361

Fat: 12g

Carbohydrates: 47g

Protein: 14g

Carrots and Tomatoes Chicken

Preparation Time: 10 Minutes

Cooking Time: 1 Hour 10 Minutes

Servings: 4

Ingredients:

- 2 pounds chicken breasts, skinless, boneless and halved
- Salt and black pepper to the taste
- 3 garlic cloves, minced
- 3 tablespoons avocado oil
- 2 shallots, chopped
- 4 carrots, sliced
- 3 tomatoes, chopped
- ¼ cup chicken stock
- 1 tablespoon Italian seasoning
- 1 tablespoon parsley, chopped

Directions:

1. Warmth up a pan through the oil over medium-high heat, add the chicken, garlic, salt and pepper and brown for 3 minutes on each side.

2. Add the rest of the fixings excluding the parsley, bring to a simmer and cook over medium-low heat for 40 minutes.

3. Add the parsley, divide the mix between plates and serve.

Nutrition:

Calories:309,

Fat:12.4,

Fiber:11.1,

Carbs:23.8,

Protein:15.3

Smoked and Hot Turkey Mix

Preparation Time: 10 Minutes

Cooking Time: 40 Minutes

Servings: 4

Ingredients:

- 1 red onion, sliced
- 1 big turkey breast, skinless, boneless and roughly cubed
- 1 tablespoon smoked paprika
- 2 chili peppers, chopped
- Salt and black pepper to the taste
- 2 tablespoons olive oil
- ½ cup chicken stock
- 1 tablespoon parsley, chopped
- 1 tablespoon cilantro, chopped

Directions:

1. Grease a roasting pan through the oil, add the turkey, onion, paprika and the rest of the ingredients, toss, introduce in the oven and bake at 425 degrees F for 40 minutes.

2. Divide the mix between plates and serve right away.

Nutrition:

Calories:310,

Fat:18.4,

Fiber:10.4,

Carbs:22.3,

Protein:33.4

Spicy Cumin Chicken

Preparation Time: 10 Minutes

Cooking Time: 25 Minutes

Servings: 4

Ingredients:

- 2 teaspoons chili powder

- 2 and ½ tablespoons olive oil

- Salt and black pepper to the taste

- 1 and ½ teaspoons garlic powder

- 1 tablespoon smoked paprika

- ½ cup chicken stock

- 1-pound chicken breasts, skinless, boneless and halved

- 2 teaspoons sherry vinegar

- 2 teaspoons hot sauce

- 2 teaspoons cumin, ground

- ½ cup black olives, pitted and sliced

Directions:

1. Warm up a pan with the oil over medium-high heat, add the chicken and brown for 3 minutes on each side.

2. Add the chili powder, salt, pepper, garlic powder and paprika, toss and cook for 4 minutes more.

3. Add the rest of the ingredients, toss, bring to a simmer and cook over medium heat for 15 minutes more.

4. Divide the mix between plates and serve.

Nutrition:

Calories:230,

Fat:18.4,

Fiber:9.4,

Carbs:15.3,

Protein:13.4

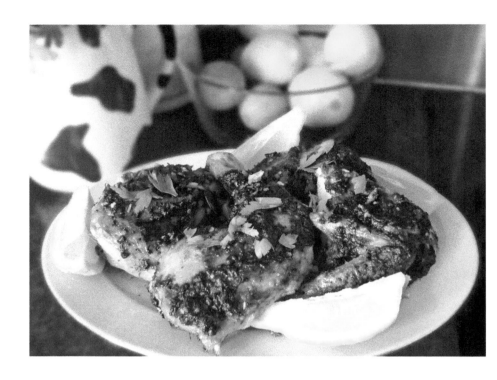

Chicken with Artichokes and Beans

Preparation Time: 10 Minutes

Cooking Time: 40 Minutes

Servings: 4

Ingredients:

- 2 tablespoons olive oil

- 2 chicken breasts, skinless, boneless and halved

- Zest of 1 lemon, grated

- 3 garlic cloves, crushed

- Juice of 1 lemon

- Salt and black pepper to the taste

- 1 tablespoon thyme, chopped

- 6 ounces canned artichokes hearts, drained

- 1 cup canned fava beans, drained and rinsed

- 1 cup chicken stock

- A pinch of cayenne pepper

- Salt and black pepper to the taste

Directions:

1. Warmth up a pan with the oil on medium-high heat, add chicken and brown for 5 minutes.

2. Add lemon juice, lemon zest, salt, pepper and the rest of the ingredients, bring to a simmer and cook over medium heat for 35 minutes.

3. Divide the mix between plates and serve right away.

Nutrition:

Calories:291,

Fat:14.9,

Fiber:10.5,

Carbs:23.8,

Protein:24.2

Chicken and Olives Tapenade

Preparation Time: 10 Minutes

Cooking Time: 25 Minutes

Servings: 4

Ingredients:

- 2 chicken breasts, boneless, skinless and halved
- 1 cup black olives, pitted
- ½ cup olive oil
- Salt and black pepper to the taste
- ½ cup mixed parsley, chopped
- ½ cup rosemary, chopped
- Salt and black pepper to the taste
- 4 garlic cloves, minced
- Juice of ½ lime

Directions:

1. In a blender, combine the olives with half of the oil and the rest of the ingredients except the chicken and pulse well.

2. Heat up a pan with the rest of the oil over medium-high heat, add the chicken and brown for 4 minutes on each side.

3. Add the olives mix, and cook for 20 minutes more tossing often.

Nutrition:

Calories:291,

Fat:12.9,

Fiber:8.5,

Carbs:15.8,

Protein:34.2

Greek Pork Chops

Preparation Time: 10 Minutes

Cooking Time: 15 Minutes

Servings: 4

Ingredients:

- 8 pork chops, boneless
- 4 teaspoon dried oregano
- 2 tablespoon Worcestershire sauce
- 3 tablespoon fresh lemon juice
- ¼ cup olive oil
- 1 teaspoon ground mustard
- 2 teaspoon garlic powder
- 2 teaspoon onion powder
- Pepper
- Salt

Directions:

1. Whisk together oil, garlic powder, onion powder, oregano, Worcestershire sauce, lemon juice, mustard, pepper, and salt.

2. Place pork chops in a baking dish then pour marinade over pork chops and coat well. Place in refrigerator overnight.

3. Preheat the grill.

4. Place pork chops on hot grill and cook for 7-8 minutes on each side.

5. Serve and enjoy.

Nutrition:

Calories 324

Fat 26.5 g

Carbohydrates 2.5 g

Sugar 1.3 g

Protein 18 g

Cholesterol 69 mg

Pork Cacciatore

Preparation Time: 10 Minutes

Cooking Time: 2 Hours

Servings: 4

Ingredients:

- 1 ½ lbs. pork chops
- 1 teaspoon dried oregano
- 1 cup beef broth
- 3 tablespoon tomato paste
- 14 oz can tomato, diced
- 2 cups mushrooms, sliced
- 1 small onion, diced
- 1 garlic clove, minced
- 2 tablespoon olive oil
- ¼ teaspoon pepper
- ½ teaspoon salt

Directions:

1. Warmth oil in a pan over medium-high heat.
2. Add pork chops in pan and cook until brown on both the sides.

3. Transfer pork chops into a pot.

4. Pour remaining ingredients over the pork chops.

5. Cover then cook on low flame for 2 hours.

6. Serve and enjoy.

Nutrition:

Calories 440

Fat 33 g

Carbohydrates 6 g

Protein 28 g

Easy Beef Kofta

Preparation Time: 10 Minutes

Cooking Time: 10 Minutes

Servings: 6

Ingredients:

- 2 lbs. ground beef
- 4 garlic cloves, minced
- 1 onion, minced
- 2 teaspoon cumin
- 1 cup fresh parsley, chopped
- ¼ teaspoon pepper
- 1 teaspoon salt
- 1 tablespoon oil

Directions:

1. With a knife, chop the beef very well.
2. Add all the fixings excluding oil into the mixing bowl and mix until combined.
3. Roll meat mixture into mini-kabab shapes.
4. Add the oil to a pan then warm up at high flame.

5. Roast the meat in the hot pan for 4-6 minutes on each side or until cooked.

6. Serve with some vegetables and a sauce if you like.

Nutrition:

Calories 223

Fat 7.3 g

Carbohydrates 2.5 g

Protein 35 g

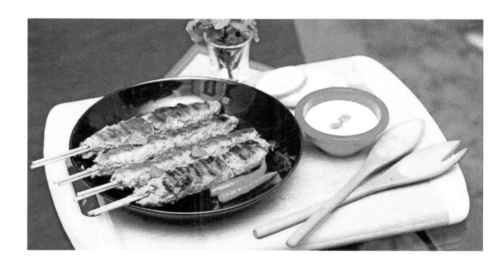

Pork with Tomato & Olives

Preparation Time: 10 Minutes

Cooking Time: 30 Minutes

Servings: 6

Ingredients:

- 6 pork chops, boneless and cut into thick slices
- 1/8 teaspoon ground cinnamon
- 1/2 cup olives, pitted and sliced
- 8 oz can tomato, crushed
- 1/4 cup beef broth
- 2 garlic cloves, chopped
- 1 large onion, sliced
- 1 tablespoon olive oil

Directions:

1. Warm up olive oil in a pan over medium heat.
2. Place pork chops in a pan and cook until lightly brown and set aside.
3. Cook garlic and onion in the same pan over medium heat, until onion is softened.
4. Add broth and bring to boil over high heat.

5. Return pork to pan and stir in crushed tomatoes and remaining ingredients.

6. Cover and simmer for 20 minutes.

7. Serve and enjoy.

Nutrition:

Calories 321

Fat 23 g

Carbohydrates 7 g

Protein 19 g

Jalapeno Lamb Patties

Preparation Time: 10 Minutes

Cooking Time: 8 Minutes

Servings: 4

Ingredients:

- 1 lb. ground lamb
- 1 jalapeno pepper, minced
- 5 basil leaves, minced
- 10 mint leaves, minced
- ¼ cup fresh parsley, chopped
- 1 cup feta cheese, crumbled
- 1 tablespoon garlic, minced
- 1 teaspoon dried oregano
- ¼ teaspoon pepper
- ½ teaspoon kosher salt

Directions:

1. Add all fixings into the mixing bowl and mix until well combined.
2. Preheat the grill to 450 F.
3. Spray grill with cooking spray.

4. Make four equal shape patties from meat mixture and place on hot grill and cook for 3 minutes. Turn patties to another side and cook for 4 minutes.

5. Serve and enjoy.

Nutrition:

Calories 317

Fat 16 g

Carbohydrates 3 g

Protein 37.5 g

Red Pepper Pork Tenderloin

Preparation Time: 10 Minutes

Cooking Time: 25 Minutes

Servings: 4

Ingredients:

- 1 lb. pork tenderloin
- 3/4 teaspoon red pepper
- 2 teaspoon dried oregano
- 1 tablespoon olive oil
- 3 tablespoon feta cheese, crumbled
- 3 tablespoon olive tapenades

Directions:

1. Add pork, oil, red pepper, and oregano in a zip-lock bag and rub well and place in a refrigerator for 2 hours.

2. Remove pork from zip-lock bag. Using sharp knife make lengthwise cut through the center of the tenderloin.

3. Spread olive tapenade on half tenderloin and sprinkle with feta cheese.

4. Fold another half of meat over to the original shape of tenderloin.

5. Tie close pork tenderloin with twine at 2-inch intervals.

6. Grill the pork tenderloin for 20 minutes.

7. Cut into slices and serve with some vegetables.

Nutrition:

Calories 215

Fat 9.1 g

Carbohydrates 1 g

Protein 30.8 g

Basil Parmesan Pork Roast

Preparation Time: 10 Minutes

Cooking Time: 2 Hours

Servings: 8

Ingredients:

- 2 lbs. lean pork roast, boneless
- 1 tablespoon parsley
- ½ cup parmesan cheese, grated
- 28 oz can tomato, diced
- 1 teaspoon dried oregano
- 1 teaspoon dried basil
- 1 teaspoon garlic powder
- Pepper
- Salt

Directions:

1. Add the meat into the crock pot.
2. Mix together tomatoes, oregano, basil, garlic powder, parsley, cheese, pepper, and salt and pour over meat.
3. Cook on low for 6 hours.
4. Serve and enjoy.

Nutrition:

Calories 294

Fat 11.6 g

Carbohydrates 5 g

Protein 38 g

Sun-dried Tomato Chuck Roast

Preparation Time: 10 Minutes

Cooking Time: 2 Hours

Servings: 6

Ingredients:

- 2 lbs. beef chuck roast
- ½ cup beef broth
- ¼ cup sun-dried tomatoes, chopped
- 25 garlic cloves, peeled
- ¼ cup olives, sliced
- 1 teaspoon dried Italian seasoning, crushed
- 2 tablespoon balsamic vinegar

Directions:

1. Place meat into a pot.
2. Pour remaining ingredients over meat.
3. Cover then cook on low flame for 2 hours.
4. Shred the meat using fork.
5. Serve and enjoy.

Nutrition:

Calories 582

Fat 43 g

Carbohydrates 5 g

Protein 40g

Lamb Stew

Preparation Time: 10 Minutes

Cooking Time: 3 Hours

Servings: 2

Ingredients:

- 1/2 lb. lamb, boneless
- 1/4 cup green olives, sliced
- 2 tablespoon lemon juice
- 1/2 onion, chopped
- 2 garlic cloves, minced
- 2 fresh thyme sprigs
- 1/4 teaspoon turmeric
- 1/2 teaspoon pepper
- 1/4 Teaspoon salt
- 1/2 teaspoon sesame seeds

Directions:

1. Slice the lamb into thin pieces.
2. Add every ingredient into a pot and stir.
3. Cover and cook on low flame for 3 hours.

4. Stir well, garnish with sesame seeds and serve.

Nutrition:

Calories 297

Fat 20.3 g

Carbohydrates 5.4 g

Protein 21 g

Lemon Lamb Leg

Preparation Time: 10 Minutes

Cooking Time: 2 Hours

Servings: 8

Ingredients:

- 4 lbs. lamb leg, boneless and slice of fat
- 1 tablespoon rosemary, crushed
- 1/4 cup water
- 1/4 cup lemon juice
- 1 teaspoon black pepper
- 1/4 teaspoon salt

Directions:

1. Place lamb into a pot.
2. Add remaining ingredients over the lamb, into the pot.
3. Cover then cook on low flame for 2 hours.
4. Remove lamb from the pot and slice it.
5. Serve and enjoy.

Nutrition:

Calories 275

Fat 10.2 g

Carbohydrates 0.4 g

Protein 42 g

Turkey and Cranberry Sauce

Preparation Time: 10 Minutes

Cooking Time: 50 Minutes

Servings: 4

Ingredients:

- 1 cup chicken stock

- 2 tablespoons avocado oil

- ½ cup cranberry sauce

- 1 big turkey breast, skinless, boneless and sliced

- 1 yellow onion, roughly chopped

- Salt and black pepper to the taste

Directions:

1. Heat up a pan with the avocado oil over medium-high heat, add the onion and sauté for 5 minutes.

2. Add the turkey and brown for 5 minutes more.

3. Add the rest of the ingredients, toss, introduce in the oven at 350 degrees F and cook for 40 minutes

Nutrition:

Calories:382,

Fat:12.6,

Fiber:9.6,

Carbs:26.6,

Protein:17.6

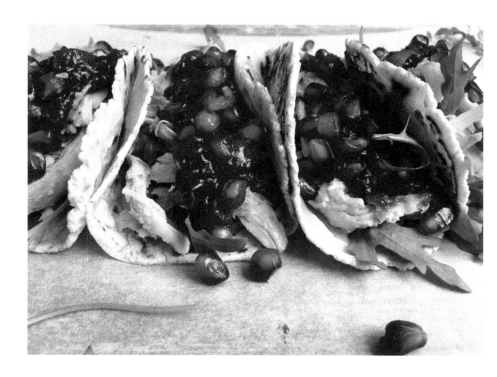

Sage Turkey Mix

Preparation Time: 10 Minutes

Cooking Time: 40 Minutes

Servings: 4

Ingredients:

- 1 big turkey breast, skinless, boneless and roughly cubed

- Juice of 1 lemon

- 2 tablespoons avocado oil

- 1 red onion, chopped

- 2 tablespoons sage, chopped

- 1 garlic clove, minced

- 1 cup chicken stock

Directions:

1. Heat up a pan with the avocado oil over medium-high heat, add the turkey and brown for 3 minutes on each side.

2. Add the rest of the fixings, let it simmer and cook over medium heat for 35 minutes.

3. Divide the mix between plates and serve with a side dish.

Nutrition:

Calories:382,

Fat:12.6,

Fiber:9.6,

Carbs:16.6,

Protein:33.2

Turkey and Asparagus Mix

Preparation Time: 10 Minutes

Cooking Time: 30 Minutes

Servings: 4

Ingredients:

- 1 bunch asparagus, trimmed and halved
- 1 big turkey breast, skinless, boneless and cut into strips
- 1 teaspoon basil, dried
- 2 tablespoons olive oil
- A pinch of salt and black pepper
- ½ cup tomato sauce
- 1 tablespoon chives, chopped

Directions:

1. Heat up a pan with the oil with medium heat, then put the turkey and brown for 4 minutes.
2. Add the asparagus and the rest of the ingredients except the chives, bring to a simmer and cook over medium heat for 25 minutes.
3. Add the chives, divide the mix between plates and serve.

Nutrition:

Calories:337,

Fat:21.2,

Fiber:10.2,

Carbs:21.4,

Protein:17.6

Herbed Almond Turkey

Preparation Time: 10 Minutes

Cooking Time: 40 Minutes

Servings: 4

Ingredients:

- 1 big turkey breast, skinless, boneless and cubed
- 1 tablespoon olive oil
- ½ cup chicken stock
- 1 tablespoon basil, chopped
- 1 tablespoon rosemary, chopped
- 1 tablespoon oregano, chopped
- 1 tablespoon parsley, chopped
- 3 garlic cloves, minced
- ½ cup almonds, toasted and chopped
- 3 cups tomatoes, chopped

Directions:

1. Warmth up a pan through the oil over medium-high heat, add the turkey and the garlic and brown for 5 minutes.

2. Add the stock in addition the rest of the fixings, bring to a simmer over medium heat and cook for 35 minutes.

3. Divide the mix between plates and serve.

Nutrition:

Calories:297,

Fat:11.2,

Fiber:9.2,

Carbs:19.4,

Protein:23.6

Thyme Chicken

Preparation Time: 10 Minutes

Cooking Time: 50 Minutes

Servings: 4

Ingredients:

- 1 tablespoon olive oil
- 4 garlic cloves, minced
- A pinch of salt and black pepper
- 2 teaspoons thyme, dried
- 12 small red potatoes, halved
- 2 pounds chicken breast, skinless, boneless and cubed
- 1 cup red onion, sliced
- ¾ cup chicken stock
- 2 tablespoons basil, chopped

Directions:

1. In a baking dish greased with the oil, add the potatoes, chicken and the rest of the ingredients, toss a bit, introduce in the oven and bake at 400 degrees F for 50 minutes.

2. Divide between plates and serve.

Nutrition:

Calories:281,

Fat:9.2,

Fiber:10.9,

Carbs:21.6,

Protein:13.6

Turkey, Artichokes and Asparagus

Preparation Time: 10 Minutes

Cooking Time: 30 Minutes

Servings: 4

Ingredients:

- 2 turkey breasts, boneless, skinless and halved
- 3 tablespoons olive oil
- 1 and ½ pounds asparagus, trimmed and halved
- 1 cup chicken stock
- A pinch of salt and black pepper
- 1 cup canned artichoke hearts, drained
- ¼ cup kalamata olives, pitted and sliced
- 1 shallot, chopped
- 3 garlic cloves, minced
- 3 tablespoons dill, chopped

Directions:

1. Warmth up a pan through the oil over medium-high heat, add the turkey and the garlic and brown for 4 minutes on each side.

2. Add the asparagus, the stock and the rest of the ingredients except the dill, bring to a simmer and cook over medium heat for 20 minutes.

3. Add the dill, divide the mix between plates and serve.

Nutrition:

Calories:291,

Fat:16,

Fiber:10.3,

Carbs:22.8,

Protein:34.5

Lemony Turkey and Pine Nuts

Preparation Time: 10 Minutes

Cooking Time: 30 Minutes

Servings: 4

Ingredients:

- 2 turkey breasts, boneless, skinless and halved
- A pinch of salt and black pepper
- 2 tablespoons avocado oil
- Juice of 2 lemons
- 1 tablespoon rosemary, chopped
- 3 garlic cloves, minced
- ¼ cup pine nuts, chopped
- 1 cup chicken stock

Directions:

1. Warmth up a pan through the oil over medium-high heat, add the garlic and the turkey and brown for 4 minutes on each side.

2. Add the rest of the fixings, let it simmer and cook over medium heat for 20 minutes.

3. Divide the mix between plates and serve with a side salad.

Nutrition:

Calories:293,

Fat:12.4,

Fiber:9.3,

Carbs:17.8,

Protein:24.5

Yogurt Chicken and Red Onion Mix

Preparation Time: 10 Minutes

Cooking Time: 30 Minutes

Servings: 4

Ingredients:

- 2 pounds chicken breast, skinless, boneless and sliced
- 3 tablespoons olive oil
- ¼ cup Greek yogurt
- 2 garlic cloves, minced
- ½ teaspoon onion powder
- A pinch of salt and black pepper
- 4 red onions, sliced

Directions:

1. In a roasting pan, combine the chicken with the oil, the yogurt and the other ingredients, introduce in the oven at 375 degrees F and bake for 30 minutes.
2. Divide chicken mix between plates and serve hot.

Nutrition:

Calories:278,

Fat:15,

Fiber:9.2,

Carbs:15.1,

Protein:23.3

Chicken and Mint Sauce

Preparation Time: 10 Minutes

Cooking Time: 30 Minutes

Servings: 4

Ingredients:

- 2 and ½ tablespoons olive oil
- 2 pounds chicken breasts, skinless, boneless and halved
- 3 tablespoons garlic, minced
- 2 tablespoons lemon juice
- 1 tablespoon red wine vinegar
- 1/3 cup Greek yogurt
- 2 tablespoons mint, chopped
- A pinch of salt and black pepper

Directions:

1. Blend the garlic plus lemon juice and the other ingredients except the oil and the chicken and pulse well.

2. Warmth up a pan through the oil over medium-high heat, add the chicken and brown for 3 minutes on each side.

3. Add the mint sauce, introduce in the oven and bake everything at 370 degrees F for 25 minutes.

4. Divide the mix between plates and serve.

Nutrition:

Calories:278,

Fat;12,

Fiber:11.2,

Carbs:18.1,

Protein:13.3

Oregano Turkey and Peppers

Preparation Time: 10 Minutes

Cooking Time: 1 Hour

Servings: 4

Ingredients:

- 2 red bell peppers, cut into strips

- 2 green bell peppers, cut into strips

- 1 red onion, chopped

- 4 garlic cloves, minced

- ½ cup black olives, pitted and sliced

- 2 cups chicken stock

- 1 big turkey breast, skinless, boneless and cut into strips

- 1 tablespoon oregano, chopped

- ½ cup cilantro, chopped

Directions:

1. In a baking pan, combine the peppers with the turkey and the rest of the ingredients, toss, introduce in the oven at 400 degrees F and roast for 1 hour.

2. Divide everything between plates and serve.

Nutrition:

Calories:229,

Fat:8.9,

Fiber:8.2,

Carbs:17.8,

Protein:33.6

Chicken and Mustard Sauce

Preparation Time: 10 Minutes

Cooking Time: 26 Minutes

Servings: 4

Ingredients:

- 1/3 cup mustard
- Salt and black pepper to the taste
- 1 red onion, chopped
- 1 tablespoon olive oil
- 1 and ½ cups chicken stock
- 4 chicken breasts, skinless, boneless, and halved
- ¼ teaspoon oregano, dried

Directions:

1. Heat up a pan with the stock over medium heat, add the mustard, onion, salt, pepper and the oregano, whisk, bring to a simmer and cook for 8 minutes.

2. Warmth up a pan through the oil over medium-high heat, add the chicken and brown for 3 minutes on each side.

3. Add chicken into the pan with the sauce, toss, simmer everything for 12 minutes more, divide between plates and serve.

Nutrition:

Calories:247,

Fat:15.1,

Fiber:9.1,

Carbs:16.6,

Protein:26.1

Chicken and Sausage Mix

Preparation Time: 10 Minutes

Cooking Time: 50 Minutes

Servings: 4

Ingredients:

- 2 zucchinis, cubed
- 1-pound Italian sausage, cubed
- 2 tablespoons olive oil
- 1 red bell pepper, chopped
- 1 red onion, sliced
- 2 tablespoons garlic, minced
- 2 chicken breasts, boneless, skinless and halved
- Salt and black pepper to the taste
- ½ cup chicken stock
- 1 tablespoon balsamic vinegar

Directions:

1. Heat up a pan with half of the oil over medium-high heat, add the sausages, brown for 3 minutes on each side and transfer to a bowl.

2. Heat up the pan again with the rest of the oil over medium-high heat, add the chicken and brown for 4 minutes on each side.

3. Return the sausage, add the rest of the ingredients as well, bring to a simmer, introduce in the oven and bake at 400 degrees F for 30 minutes.

4. Divide everything between plates and serve.

Nutrition:

Calories:293,

Fat:13.1,

Fiber:8.1,

Carbs:16.6,

Protein:26.1

Coriander and Coconut Chicken

Preparation Time: 10 Minutes

Cooking Time: 30 Minutes

Servings: 4

Ingredients:

- 2 pounds chicken thighs, skinless, boneless and cubed
- 2 tablespoons olive oil
- Salt and black pepper to the taste
- 3 tablespoons coconut flesh, shredded
- 1 and ½ teaspoons orange extract
- 1 tablespoon ginger, grated
- ¼ cup orange juice
- 2 tablespoons coriander, chopped
- 1 cup chicken stock
- ¼ teaspoon red pepper flakes

Directions:

1. Warmth up a pan through the oil over medium-high heat, add the chicken and brown for 4 minutes on each side.

2. Add salt, pepper and the rest of the ingredients, bring to a simmer and cook over medium heat for 20 minutes.

3. Divide the mix between plates and serve hot.

Nutrition:

Calories:297,

Fat:14.4,

Fiber:9.6,

Carbs:22,

Protein:25

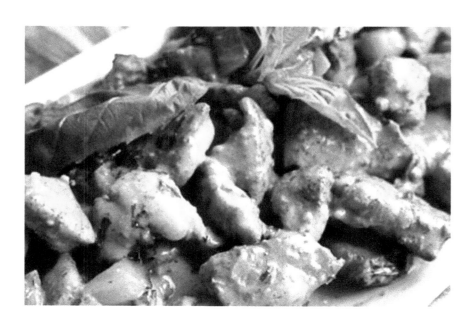

Saffron Chicken Thighs and Green Beans

Preparation Time: 10 Minutes

Cooking Time: 25 Minutes

Servings: 4

Ingredients:

- 2 pounds chicken thighs, boneless and skinless

- 2 teaspoons saffron powder

- 1-pound green beans, trimmed and halved

- ½ cup Greek yogurt

- Salt and black pepper to the taste

- 1 tablespoon lime juice

- 1 tablespoon dill, chopped

Directions:

1. In a roasting pan, combine the chicken with the saffron, green beans and the rest of the ingredients, toss a bit, introduce in the oven and bake at 400 degrees F for 25 minutes.

2. Divide everything between plates and serve.

Nutrition:

Calories:274,

Fat:12.3,

Fiber:5.3,

Carbs:20.4,

Protein:14.3

Chicken and Olives Salsa

Preparation Time: 10 Minutes

Cooking Time: 25 Minutes

Servings: 4

Ingredients:

- 2 tablespoon avocado oil
- 4 chicken breast halves, skinless and boneless
- Salt and black pepper to the taste
- 1 tablespoon sweet paprika
- 1 red onion, chopped
- 1 tablespoon balsamic vinegar
- 2 tablespoons parsley, chopped
- 1 avocado, peeled, pitted and cubed
- 2 tablespoons black olives, pitted and chopped

Directions:

1. Heat up your grill over medium-high heat, add the chicken brushed with half of the oil and seasoned with paprika, salt and pepper, cook for 7 minutes on each side and divide between plates.

2. Meanwhile, in a bowl, mix the onion with the rest of the ingredients and the remaining oil, toss, add on top of the chicken and serve.

Nutrition:

Calories:289,

Fat:12.4,

Fiber:9.1,

Carbs:23.8,

Protein:14.3

Lemon and Garlic Fettucine

Preparation Time: 5 Minutes

Cooking Time: 15 Minutes

Servings: 5

Ingredients:

- 8 ounces of whole wheat fettuccine
- 4 tablespoons of extra virgin olive oil
- 4 cloves of minced garlic
- 1 cup of fresh breadcrumbs
- ¼ cup of lemon juice
- 1 teaspoon of freshly ground pepper
- ½ teaspoon of salt
- 2 cans of 4 ounce boneless and skinless sardines (dipped in tomato sauce)
- ½ cup of chopped up fresh parsley
- ¼ cup of finely shredded Parmesan cheese

Directions:

1. Take a large-sized pot and bring water to a boil.
2. Cook pasta for 10 minutes until Al Dente.

3. Take a small-sized skillet and place it over medium heat.

4. Add 2 tablespoons of oil and allow it to heat up.

5. Add garlic and cook for 20 seconds.

6. Transfer the garlic to a medium-sized bowl

7. Add breadcrumbs to the hot skillet and cook for 5-6 minutes until golden

8. Whisk in lemon juice, pepper and salt into the garlic bowl

9. Add pasta to the bowl (with garlic) and sardines, parsley and Parmesan

10. Stir well and sprinkle bread crumbs

11. Enjoy!

Nutrition:

Calories: 480

Fat: 21g

Carbohydrates: 53g

Protein: 23g

Roasted Broccoli with Parmesan

Preparation Time: 10 Minutes

Cooking Time: 10 Minutes

Servings: 4

Ingredients:

- 2 head broccolis, cut into florets
- 2 tablespoons extra-virgin olive oil
- 2 teaspoons garlic, minced
- Zest of 1 lemon
- Pinch of salt
- ½ cup Parmesan cheese, grated

Directions:

1. Pre-heat your oven to 400 degrees Fahrenheit.
2. Take a large bowl and add broccoli with 2 tablespoons olive oil, lemon zest, garlic, lemon juice and salt.
3. Spread mix on the baking sheet in single layer and sprinkle with Parmesan cheese.
4. Bake for 10 minutes until tender.
5. Transfer broccoli to serving the dish.

6. Serve and enjoy!

Nutrition:

Calories: 154

Fat: 11g

Carbohydrates: 10g

Protein: 9g

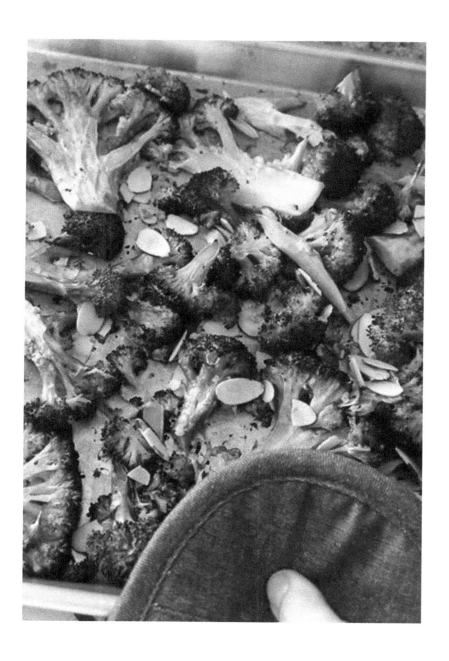

Spinach and Feta Bread

Preparation Time: 10 Minutes

Cooking Time: 12 Minutes

Servings: 6

Ingredients:

- 6 ounces of sun-dried tomato pesto
- 6 pieces of 6-inch whole wheat pita bread
- 2 chopped up Roma plum tomatoes
- 1 bunch of rinsed and chopped spinach
- 4 sliced fresh mushrooms
- ½ cup of crumbled feta cheese
- 2 tablespoons of grated Parmesan cheese
- 3 tablespoons of olive oil
- Ground black pepper as needed

Directions:

1. Pre-heat your oven to 350 degrees Fahrenheit.

2. Spread your tomato pesto onto one side of your pita bread and place on your baking sheet (with the pesto side up).

3. Top up the pitas with spinach, tomatoes, feta cheese, mushrooms and Parmesan cheese.

4. Drizzle with some olive oil and season nicely with pepper.

5. Bake in your oven for around 12 minutes until the breads are crispy.

6. Cut up the pita into quarters and serve!

Nutrition:

Calories: 350

Fat: 17g

Carbohydrates: 41g

Protein:11g

Quick Zucchini Bowl

Preparation Time: 10 Minutes

Cooking Time: 10 Minutes

Servings: 4

Ingredients:

- ½ pound of pasta
- 2 tablespoons of olive oil
- 6 crushed garlic cloves
- 1 teaspoon of red chili
- 2 finely sliced spring onions
- 3 teaspoons of chopped rosemary
- 1 large zucchini cut up in half, lengthways and sliced
- 5 large portabella mushrooms
- 1 can of tomatoes
- 4 tablespoons of Parmesan cheese
- Fresh ground black pepper

Directions:

1. Cook the pasta.
2. Take a large-sized frying pan and place over medium heat.

3. Add oil and allow the oil to heat up.

4. Add garlic, onion and chili and sauté for a few minutes until golden.

5. Add zucchini, rosemary and mushroom and sauté for a few minutes.

6. Increase the heat to medium-high and add tinned tomatoes to the sauce until thick.

7. Drain your boiled pasta and transfer to a serving platter.

8. Pour the tomato mix on top and mix using tongs.

9. Garnish with Parmesan cheese and freshly ground black pepper.

10. Enjoy!

Nutrition:

Calories: 361

Fat: 12g

Carbohydrates: 47g

Protein: 14g

Healthy Basil Platter

Preparation Time: 25 Minutes

Cooking Time: 15 Minutes

Servings: 4

Ingredients:

- 2 pieces of red pepper seeded and cut up into chunks

- 2 pieces of red onion cut up into wedges

- 2 mild red chilies, diced and seeded

- 3 coarsely chopped garlic cloves

- 1 teaspoon of golden caster sugar

- 2 tablespoons of olive oil (plus additional for serving)

- 2 pounds of small ripe tomatoes quartered up

- 12 ounces of dried pasta

- Just a handful of basil leaves

- 2 tablespoons of grated Parmesan

Directions:

1. Pre-heat the oven to 392 degrees Fahrenheit.

2. Take a large-sized roasting tin and scatter pepper, red onion, garlic and chilies.

3. Sprinkle sugar on top.

4. Drizzle olive oil then season with pepper and salt.

5. Roast the veggies in your oven for 15 minutes.

6. Take a large-sized pan and cook the pasta in boiling, salted water until Al Dente.

7. Drain them.

8. Remove the veggies from the oven and tip in the pasta into the veggies.

9. Toss well and tear basil leaves on top.

10. Sprinkle Parmesan and enjoy!

Nutrition:

Calories: 452

Fat: 8g

Carbohydrates: 88g

Protein: 14g

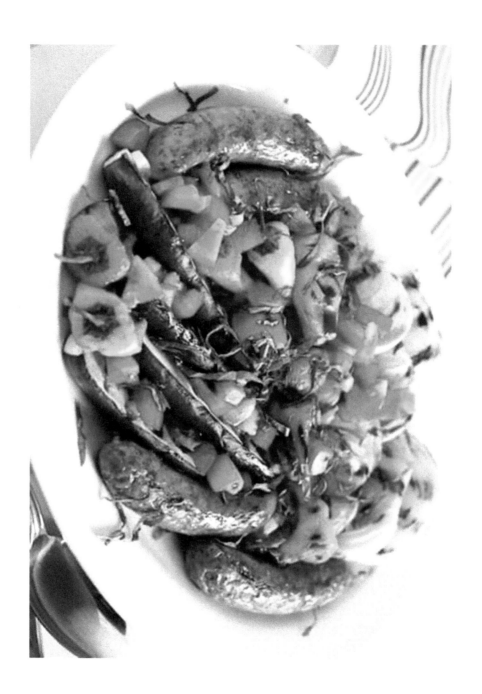

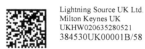